Contents

Preface

If you have already attempted to stop smoking cigarettes, then you are well aware of how difficult it is to rid your life of this pernicious habit. Why do people continue smoking cigarettes even though they're aware of the negatives? Is it the power of nicotine that keeps smokers hooked? Are they afraid of gaining weight? Are they waiting until after the holidays? Is it that smokers simply say, *"I'm going to quit soon,"* purely out of guilt or shame yet don't have any real intention of quitting? Are smokers even to blame for the addiction? If you want to quit smoking cigarettes, or drop any toxic and deadly addiction for that matter, then start with understanding and observing your mind.

If you're a smoker, this 30-day mindfulness program will help you approach quitting from a different perspective. You have nothing to lose by attempting this short mindfulness program and you can even use our exercises along with other methods of quitting. Quitting smoking may seem like an impossible feat, but there are reasons for this misperception. Smoking has a lot more to do with conditioning than it does with inhaling tobacco smoke, the effects of nicotine, or taste.

The following pages involve a 30-day program made up of lessons and exercises to help you overcome thought patterns, feelings, and behaviors that have kept you in the cigarette trap. Though these lessons and exercises can be applied to any adverse reliance, this program will focus specifically on the problem of smoking cigarettes.

For some readers, they'll overcome quickly and will drop the unhealthy thoughts and habits in no time; and for others, they'll overcome gradually. In either case, if you stick with the program, you'll start to witness your dependency on cigarettes weaken. Don't critique your progress, as this isn't a competition and there isn't a goal you must attain. Let the habitual thoughts, feelings, and dependency simply drop as you work through the exercises and lessons.

It's not necessary to complete these days in order, nor should you be religious about completing them successfully. There is no such thing as a successful completion of this program. The bottom line is to observe and awaken, and that cannot be obtained through success, force, pressure, struggle, or competition. Simply relax, follow the program, and the grip of cigarettes can loosen.

You'll also notice that mindfulness, silence, and stillness are a regular discipline for each day. Because you've been influenced by a dependency-based society that demands instant gratification, silence and stillness may seem nearly impossible for you to practice. For this reason, we'll incorporate this discipline from the outset. A quiet and still mind is an incredibly powerful resource, but one that requires daily maintenance.

It should also be noted that you're not required to quit smoking during this program. The point being: by practicing the following exercises and lessons in the days to come, you won't even need willpower to stop. With that said, it's not encouraged that you smoke, just that you do not attempt to force quit. "Force quitting" rarely works for the long-term.

One of the most important lessons to keep in mind is to not fight the addiction while participating in this program. Dependencies, habits, and strong patterns of thinking are empowered by a fight and struggle. You can smoke for the length of this program without regret or remorse; unless you witness the habit drop – then let it go and never pick it up again. Smoking, like most unhealthy habits, feeds on negative thought patterns, fear, and struggle. This program will help you overcome without a conflict.

You'll need about 15-30 minutes per day for the program, but feel free to spend more time if needed. The amount of time doesn't matter, as long as you're in an environment that allows you to concentrate without distraction.

One last thing: If you're like most people, you might dependent on caffeine or alcohol to some extent. If you are, do your best to lessen the consumption of these substances over the next 30 days. Can you cut consumption of these substances in half, or more? It's important that your mind is sober and your body relaxed to make the most of these exercises.

Let's get started.

Day 1

Exercise:

Find a place without distraction, and turn off all electronics. Sit with your back straight, kneel, or lie on a hard surface (not bed) and remain in silence for 10 minutes.

During these 10 minutes, take deep and focused breaths and hold them for a few seconds each. Exhale slowly. Listen intently to your breathing. Don't try to change it – simply listen, and feel the air go in and out.

*When you're ready, repeat the mantra: **"Be still. Be silent."** Repeat this slowly multiple times out loud as well as quietly. You might experience boredom or anxiety, but continue repeating the mantra regardless. Repeat it until you're calm and focused. You can continue the deep breathing during the mantra, or take deep breaths during pauses. Don't rush.*

Each of the 30 days will have this time of silence, focused breathing, and a mantra. Except for this page, the end of each day will remind you of the minutes you are to spend in silence and focused breathing; and will also have a mantra for you to practice. You can repeat the mantras during your times of silence and focused breathing, or following. Remember, there is no right or wrong way to do this.

Long-held beliefs, thoughts, and feelings will often fight change; in fact, they're energized by fighting. Instead of fighting the old ideas and thoughts about smoking *(i.e. what you believe cigarettes do for you)*, meet them with silence and observation. Let the exercises and lessons in this program guide you.

(Share this experience using **#30DaysBreathing**)

<u>Day 2</u>

Exercise:

Ponder this question: Can you remember a point in your life when you did not want, need, or depend on cigarettes, even the slightest bit?

Writing is extremely beneficial to the mind; especially when pondering. Write down your thoughts about this particular question. If your mind drifts, then write whatever thoughts emerge. It's okay if you have nothing to write, but ponder the question regardless.

Were you able to remember a period in your life when you were completely free from smoking cigarettes? If you're like many people, you may have to return to memories of childhood to determine that period. It's not uncommon for a person to experience a conditioned belief about smoking early on and continue experiencing its influence throughout life. We're taught early, in culture and family, to identify cigarettes with specific advantages (*i.e. relaxation, maturity, popularity, etc*); and as a result, an attachment to a false belief and dangerous habit is born.

Recognize that your beliefs about cigarettes are learned. However, they can be dropped quickly and completely; and you have the capability to drop. In other words, you are not controlled, identified, or dominated by a learned misconception of cigarettes. You may be living with conflicting ideas about smoking; however, such conditioned and strong beliefs can be unlearned. Discover that cigarettes have no power or influence over you.

*10 minutes of silence and focused breathing. Repeat the mantra: **"Drop. Unlearn. Discover."**

(Share this experience using **#30DaysPonder**)

<u>Day 3</u>

Exercise:

For this exercise, you can use paper and pen, but simply sitting and pondering for a while may suffice. Identify all of the associations tied to cigarettes in your life. Though not necessary, it may be best to write down everything that comes to mind. For example, a person may reflect deeply and determine that smoking is associated, directly or indirectly, with friendship, stress relief, or work. Become keenly aware of the associations. Take as much time as is needed to identify the connections to smoking cigarettes.

Think like a detective for this exercise: What connection does smoking have with your environment, work, social circle, family, habits, upbringing, cultural conditioning, fears, aspirations, etc? See smoking not as individualistic (*i.e. as something that defines "you"*) but as dependent and connected to other things. Identify and observe the associations. However, be careful not to blame the associations. Neither shame yourself, nor blame the associations...just identify and observe them. For example, your job, family, or friends are not to blame for your habit.

If you commit to practicing this exercise often, you'll begin to see the connections in real-time (*here and now*) and will awaken to the truth that a deadly smoking habit has a lot of help. What should you do about those associations? You'll know what to do once you have identified and observed them thoroughly.

*10 minutes of silence and focused breathing. Repeat the mantra: **"I accept positive connections. I let go of the negative."**

(Share this experience using **#30DaysAssociation**)

<u>Day 4</u>

Exercise:

Close your eyes, take a deep breath, hold the breath for a few seconds, and then imagine a colorful plume of air being exhaled from your lungs and filling the area around you. You can imagine any color plume you wish. Repeat this at least three times.

We are creative beings. One of the reasons people attach to cigarettes is the large, impressive, and cool looking plume of smoke that is exhaled. For many people who smoke, it becomes sort of an art form – they exhale in their unique own way and can see the smoke fill the area and drift away. There's a mystique to smoking that is undeniable – imagine smoking cigarettes without the smoke. Unaware of it, you are attaching to a creative process and developing your own style of smoking. However, it's important that you awaken and see past this apparent mystique.

Even though the smoke plume can appear creative and impressive, it is only a cloud made of tobacco and toxins. To detach from this ingenious dependency, practice imagining the most beautiful plumes of clean air being exhaled from your lungs. Use the power of your imagination to detach from smoking. Don't let the tobacco industry and its corporations manipulate your imagination, habits, health, mind, and breathing. There is nothing special about the smoke.

*10 minutes of silence and focused breathing. Repeat the mantra: **"My breath is clean and pure."**

(Share this experience using **#30DaysPlume**)

Day 5

Exercise:

Count to 25 slowly, pausing for a few seconds before the next number; then, count backward from 25 slowly. Try this with your eyes closed. While counting up you can imagine yourself being lifted into the sky; and then while counting down, descending back to earth.

Our world today is about speed. Everyone seems to be in a rush, yet most people are unsatisfied; and, they have no clue where they're going. Chasing the next best thing is a fruitless endeavor. It's the rare person who slows down to enjoy the present moment, regardless of its nature. Because there seem to be so many problems, and most jobs are focused on resolving those problems, people are compelled to accept anxiety and rush toward a reward and conclusion. That surely isn't happiness. Happiness can only be found in the present moment, not in a hypothetical future of rewards and successes. Rushing is another form of going nowhere.

How many times have you used cigarettes to launch you forward and get things done, or to relax and recharge? This is destructive to your peace of mind and health: concentration suffers, stress levels rise, and awareness to the present moment isn't possible. Smoking is not a healthy boost for getting work done or recharging.

It's critical to slow down. You only have one life to live – don't rush through it, and don't be dependent on anything that encourages you to rush. Be still, and slow down.

*10 minutes of silence and focused breathing. Repeat the mantra: **"Slow down. Do not rush. Enjoy the present moment."**

(Share this experience using **#30DaysCount**)

<u>Day 6</u>

Exercise:

On a piece of paper, write down all the labels and adjectives that you and others use to identify you.

For example, do you see yourself as a son, daughter, mother, father, student, teacher, cashier, friend, engineer, accountant, employee, employer, roommate, husband, wife, etc? And what adjectives do you use to label yourself; for example, do you identify yourself as addicted, failed, successful, happy, depressed, good, moral, unethical, lustful, greedy, valuable, worthless, etc? Don't only write down the labels and descriptions you perceive, but also write down what you believe others label you as: do you believe others see you as a valuable friend, stupid and incompetent employee, a smoking addict, extremely smart and talented worker, etc? Take as long as you need, and fill up a sheet of paper with those labels and descriptions.

After you've done that, tear the paper into multiple pieces and throw it away. Those labels and adjectives mean nothing. They're not *you*. You cannot be defined, labeled, described, or controlled by titles. Most people poison their conscience with such learned vocabulary. They blindly believe these words hold power – they'll even fight, stress out, become ill, and die to make these words part of reality. Cigarettes teach you to identify with particular words, which are only thoughts. Unlearn them. In other words, you are not an addict or an unhealthy person. You are simply *you* without the desire or need to poison yourself with cigarettes. You do not need to smoke to identify.

*10 minutes of silence and focused breathing. Repeat the mantra: **"I am not a label, title, or description."**

(Share this experience using **#30DaysIdentity**)

Day 7

Exercise:

Find a hard object that you can hold in the palm of your hand (such as a stone, ball, or bottle). With either hand, grip this object tightly and squeeze it as hard as you can. Squeeze it forcefully until you can't hold onto it any longer. Drop the object when ready.

If you could continue squeezing that object forever, perhaps you would; but your muscles and nerves can only endure for so long. At some point, you simply and quickly release the grip and drop the object. There isn't a process to the drop; it just happens when your body says that's enough. The release happens naturally without effort.

Letting go of an unhealthy dependency, habit, thought pattern, addiction, emotion, or behavior can be that easy. Letting go can be as natural and guilt-free as dropping the object you were gripping onto so tightly in this exercise; so, take a lesson from your body's experience. When it's time to let go, then let go.

The time to let go of smoking is always...now. Just let the drop happen, because you have the knowledge and awareness to see that your body and mind have no beneficial use for cigarettes, despite its prevalence in society. Just because the people around you are unable to let go of a toxic dependency, doesn't mean you have an obligation to hold onto it. There is no legitimate, good, or beneficial reason to smoke.

*10 minutes of silence and focused breathing. Repeat the mantra: **"Letting go is natural. I can let go, here and now."**

(Share this experience using **#30DaysGrip**)

<u>Day 8</u>

Exercise:

Deliberately feel the sensation of water on your skin for at least 5 minutes. You can do this exercise in the shower, while washing your wands, taking a bath, going for a swim, walking in the rain, or simply placing your hand in a sink filled with water. Close your eyes if you like.

How often do you deliberately experience the essence of water? We take it for granted every day. It's a remarkable chemical substance in the universe that is necessary for all life. Without it, we wouldn't exist. This one transparent and fluid substance has immense capacity. A large percentage of your physical body is made of this natural substance. Experience it.

Every day we jump in the shower, wash our hands, and drink it – but rarely do we take time to slowly and deliberately appreciate our natural response to water. Cigarettes can never give you the energy, sensation, reality, and present moment awareness that water can give. Water is an example of a positive dependency that doesn't bind you emotionally or spiritually; smoking, on the other hand, binds you to an unhealthy habit with terrible long term consequences.

There are many lessons that water can teach: fluidity, flow, evaporation, change, motion, stillness, and life. You can't get any of those lessons through smoking or any hazardous habit for that matter.

*10 minutes of silence and focused breathing. Repeat the mantra: **"I am fluid. I change. I flow."**

(Share this experience using **#30DaysWater**)

<u>Day 9</u>

Exercise:

For 5 minutes, hum to yourself with mouth and eyes closed. Take deep breaths between pauses. You can do this exercise lying on a hard floor, standing, kneeling, or sitting with back straight.

This exercise may seem cliché, but there is a lot that can be learned from the sound of your voice during a long hum. Humming relaxes the body and mind – similar to listening to raindrops, crickets in the evening, leaves rustling, or a waterfall. It is believed the reason for this relaxing effect involves the wavelengths produced and sent in perpetual flow.

But what's especially interesting about your humming is that it's directly related to your breathing. If you take shorter, rushed breaths, your hum won't be as long and effective; but if you take concentrated, deep breaths, then your hum will serve to relax your body, and possibly bring you into present moment awareness. Also, did you notice that it was *you* who was relaxing *you*? You weren't dependent on smoking a cigarette to become calm and still. Without smoking, you have the ability to calm yourself.

From time to time, listen to yourself hum; listen to the wavelengths you produce from your own being. This is always available to you in the present moment.

*10 minutes of silence and focused breathing. Repeat the mantra: **"Calmness and stillness are always present."**

(Share this experience using **#30DaysHum**)

Day 10

Exercise:

On a piece of paper (any size) write down the goals that you've been striving to achieve – i.e. the goals that you believe will bring you fulfillment. For example: a new job, a house in a nice neighborhood, traveling the world, a business, a family, new friends, a degree or certification, building a network, reaching a net worth of a million dollars, etc.

Now, tear up the paper into multiple pieces and throw away.

Goals can be very helpful and useful if they're not obsessed over. However, in the modern world people develop a reliance on goals. Think about all the times you've said something like, *"I need to quit soon," "I must reach this," "I'll do anything to accomplish that"*, etc. It's often the case that people spend more time worrying about their goals, than freely doing something in the present moment to reach them. Plus, the goal in itself is fleeting, while the journey in the present moment is real and lasting.

The habit of thinking that goals must be met, or else failure ensues, is subtly fixed to dependencies. When you've attempted to quit smoking in the past, what was the goal? What was it that you felt you needed to achieve? Did you attach your worth to the accomplishment of that goal? You don't need to reach a goal to quit smoking...you can quit now.

*10 minutes of silence and focused breathing. Repeat the mantra: **"My happiness does not depend on meeting a goal. I'm happy now."***

(Share this experience using **#30DaysGoals**)

<u>Day 11</u>

Exercise:

Pinch the skin on the back of your hand or forearm until there is discomfort and slight pain. It's not necessary to pinch hard enough to bruise yourself, just enough to feel a small burn.

Did I cause the pain by asking you to do this exercise? No; you caused this pain to yourself – think about this carefully. You even decided how much pain to give yourself, and when to relieve the pain. You can't blame me or anyone else for the pain you just experienced. You were solely responsible. You were also responsible for letting go.

This is easily understood with regard to physical pain, such as pinching oneself; however, we have a lot of difficulties understanding this lesson as it applies to adverse emotions and feelings. How often have you said, and have heard others say, *"He makes me so angry when…"*, *"I'm depressed because she…"*, or *"I'm so frustrated that they…"* No person ever makes you experience negative feelings. It's always you who are experiencing them; and then placing the blame on others. Essentially, you are emotionally pinching yourself and not letting go.

People go their entire lives without releasing the pinch while using cigarettes to cope with the pain. Instead of letting go, they scream at others, *"Release the pain! Let go! Fix this! Stop this! You're to blame!"* Wake up and see that you are solely responsible for letting go of the pain, and you can do it now, without the use of cigarettes.

*10 minutes of silence and focused breathing. Repeat the mantra: **"I can release negative feelings, here and now."***

(Share this experience using **#30DaysPinch**)

Day 12

Exercise:

Spend 5 minutes smelling something aromatic: a piece of fruit, a spice, tea, pine, cedar, a flower, a scented candle, etc. Focus on the smell of that one thing for the entire 5 minutes. Don't let anything distract you from the smell.

How often do you take time to enjoy a fragrant smell? One of the lies of modern society is that if you stop and enjoy your five senses for too long, you'll miss out on…fill in the blank. While people are rushing toward their goals with stress levels spiking, they're totally missing out on awareness in the present moment. People stare at images of food that others have posted on the internet, but don't take the time to smell or taste real food in the present moment.

What's better: inhaling toxic cigarette smoke and smelling like a chimney, or enjoying the smell of vanilla, orange, or pine in the present moment? The first is fake and illusory; the second is real and sensational. Smoking does a great job of stealing time and energy from your other senses, such as smell. One of the best ways to get into the present moment and away from an illusion is through focusing on smell and the use of your other senses. Don't let smoking diminish your other senses any longer. Awaken your sense of smell.

*10 minutes of silence and focused breathing. Repeat the mantra: ***"I can sense the present."***

(Share this experience using **#30DaysAroma**)

<u>Day 13</u>

Exercise:

On a sheet of paper (any size) write down all the internal lies that you regularly hear about yourself – i.e. within your mind.

Now, tear the paper into multiple pieces, and throw away.

It's common to have an internal voice (or voices) within your mind, playing a record of lies over and over. We eventually begin to accept these lies and let them impact our growth and happiness. Most people you see daily have these recurring internal voices, and most people are oblivious to them – sort of like white noise. This isn't a mental illness, but a way in which the mind works. We all experience these internal quiet voices whispering untruths about our being. These lies are nothing to fear, but they need to be observed. Writing them down can help you observe and become aware of their deceptions.

The power of silence, focused breathing, and mantras, which you have been practicing, is to draw out the lies. Let them manifest, and observe them. Common internal lies include: *"You are a loser, you'll never quit smoking," "You have become nothing, and you will never improve," "You are worthless. No one likes you," "You'll always be alone," "You're a burden,"* and so on. These thoughts are not part of you; however, the deception is to make you believe they are. Like many things in our culture, bad habits, such as smoking, implant many of these lies clandestinely.

*10 minutes of silence and focused breathing. Repeat the mantra: ***"Thoughts are only thoughts - nothing more."***

(Share this experience using **#30DaysLies**)

Day 14

Exercise:

Say the words "Guilt", "Shame", and "Regret" 10 times to yourself out loud. Don't rush. Pause between each repetition. For the pause, you can take a deep breath. Your eyes can remain open or closed. Again, don't rush - say the words slowly and observe any thoughts, feelings, or images that emerge internally.

Now, say these words again 10 times, but with a smile.

What futile credence we give words such as Guilt, Shame, and Regret. We use these words on ourselves as well as others; they become regular vocabulary for our internal recurring voices. And in the end, they're mere words that hold no power. What would these words be without a facial expression, tone, inflection, or emphasis?

When you said these three specific words, what thoughts came to mind, what did you feel, and was there a reaction in your body? If there is a reaction, such as shortness of breath or a frown, people tend to interpret it as sadness; but this reaction is a learned behavior. We've been taught to feel and think a certain way concerning guilt, shame, and regret. The truth is: these words mean nothing.

Smoking, like most toxic dependencies, flourishes on these three words and the learned reactions they produce. But see them for what they are…mere words with no power. Don't let guilt, shame, or regret influence you to smoke.

*10 minutes of silence and focused breathing. Repeat the mantra: ***"I am not Guilt. I am not Shame. I am not Regret."***

(Share this experience using **#30DaysGSR**)

<u>Day 15</u>

Exercise:

This exercise may be the most dreaded because few people enjoy cold showers until they see the light. Yes, it's time to take a cold shower – in fact; hopefully, you'll take many from now on. The benefits are awesome.

Simply put, take a cold shower. Don't even touch the hot water handle or knob. If you have never taken a cold shower, or if it's been some time, start by turning on the water before stepping into the shower, let the water hit your hands or feet first, and then gradually step into the stream. If you find this especially difficult at first, splash the cold water on your face before stepping into the stream. If needed, count to 20 or 30 before turning off the shower or switching to warm. You'll discover your own way.

As mentioned in other exercises, try not to make this a competition. The purpose is to observe yourself before, during, and after the cold shower; as well as to focus on your breathing. You'll find deep breaths during the cold shower will make the experience much more tolerable. People who start taking cold showers typically don't enjoy them until they've gone a few weeks enduring one or two a day. After a short time, they begin to see awesome benefits to their breathing, awareness, and stress reduction. You may even want to practice a mantra while taking a cold shower – that would be great for focusing the mind. If you're ever tempted to smoke, jump in a cold shower!

*15 minutes of silence and focused breathing. Repeat the mantra: **"I accept this moment. I can endure. I am alive."**

(Share this experience using **#30DaysColdShower**)

Day 16

Exercise:

Choose an object that you use and rely on every day and that you sometimes lose – such as a key, cell phone, pen, hat, toothbrush, or television controller.

Now, attempt to lose this object. Hide it well, and try to make yourself forget where it is.

More than likely you won't be able to lose this object, as hard as you try, because you have applied a lot of attention to the process of losing it and trying to make yourself forget. At this point, losing it is nearly impossible. Why do you think this is?

If you try to drop a dependency, behavior, thought pattern, addiction, or any unhealthy vice using a lot of thought, attention, focus, struggle, and effort… you'll never lose it. It will be with you in one form or another for a very long time, possibly forever. The point is: whatever you give attention to consistently, will be difficult to lose. This is the reason why people become anxious when attempting to follow a strict program – they can't stop giving thought and attention to the problems they're fighting. These problems eventually become an intimate part of their lives. Remember, rival enemies maintain a devoted relationship.

People have indeed given up smoking by identifying as an addict and following a plan. Though that may be an effective approach, many of these people continue to battle with smoking in thought and attention. Allow it to be lost.

*15 minutes of silence and focused breathing. Repeat the mantra: **"I do not need to hold on. I allow it to be lost."**

(Share this experience using **#30DaysLose**)

<u>Day 17</u>

Exercise:

Go out and buy a small trash can. You should be able to find one cheaply. If you don't have the funds for this exercise, you can use an empty box or container; however, a small trash can works better for its symbolism.

Designate this specific trash can your "concerns and worries can" (or use any title you wish) – some people benefit from writing this label directly onto the can.

Now, write down (on scraps of paper or whatever paper you wish to use) any concerns, worries, and adverse thoughts that you may be experiencing today, and throw them into the can. Try to practice this every day: quickly write down worries, concerns, and negative thoughts, and then throw them into the can. It may be beneficial to have a supply of scrap paper near the can for easy access.

This exercise may seem simple, but let's go beyond throwing your written concerns, worries, and thoughts away. Designate a few times during the week for sifting through the can and taking out random worries and concerns from days prior – just reach in and pull some out. Observe them, but don't judge yourself. This is a great exercise to learn your negative thought patterns and the lies that grip your conscience. If you stick with this practice, you may gain a deeper understanding and realization into the dependencies, habits, thought patterns, and feelings that have been exacerbated or supported by smoking.

*"*15 minutes of silence and focused breathing. Repeat the mantra: ***"There is nothing to worry about. All is well."***

(Share this experience using **#30DaysTrash**)

Day 18

Exercise:

Taste something by eating it very slowly for at least 5 minutes. Pick something with a lot of flavor: a piece of fruit, a strong tea, a spice, soup with many ingredients, honey, etc. Close your eyes through most of your tasting. Savor the piece of food slowly. Pay close attention to the feel of the taste on your tongue. Chew slowly.

Cigarettes do a great job of stealing presence away from the other senses, as do many dependencies. Since cigarettes are directly related to neurochemicals, the more those senses are abused the more our other senses are neglected, such as taste. When was the last time you thoroughly enjoyed the taste of grapes, honey, dark chocolate, olive oil, or cheese? I don't mean enjoying the flavor for a few seconds and then continuing to eat, but to let the flavor linger before taking another bite.

The taste of pineapple, pepper, mango, or apple is far more real and satisfying than a cigarette. It may sound silly to say that, but it's true, because those foods are based in reality, whereas the taste of tobacco is masked by the carcinogens and flavor additives. You can genuinely interact with real food in the present moment, and it won't hypnotize you into an illusory relationship like cigarettes purpose to do.

Let the taste of real food, flavors, and spices bring you into the present moment. You won't miss the illusory taste of cigarettes. Don't be fooled any longer by fake tastes.

*15 minutes of silence and focused breathing. Repeat the mantra: **"I am free to taste."**

(Share this experience using **#30DaysTaste**)

Day 19

Exercise:

Observe your body. Observe how it feels, moves, and reacts. More direction is explained below.

If you're still smoking cigarettes, observe your body movements, sounds, sensations, and breaths during the habit. Do you talk differently? Do you move fast or slow? How is your heartbeat? How is your posture? What is your breathing like? Where do you tend to look? Try to observe everything about your body if you are still smoking. Be aware of the cigarette's effect on your body.

If you have dropped the attachment to smoking, then continue with the 15 minutes of silence and focused breathing, but get in touch with your body. A good way to do this is by touching each body part and saying its name, leaving your hand on the part for a few seconds and feeling its texture and warmth. Start with your head: place your hand on your head and say, *"I am touching my head."* And then work your way down to your shoulders, arms, stomach, legs, knees, and feet. Focus your attention on one body part at a time. Say its name and describe what you are touching.

*15 minutes of silence and focused breathing. Repeat the mantra: **"I am not my body."**

(Share this experience using **#30DaysBody**)

Day 20

Exercise:

Using objects that can stack (rocks, books, boxes, containers, pillows, etc), stack them slowly and carefully until they fall.

When the stack collapses, smile and laugh.

The lives of many people are spent stacking things for the goal of success, as defined by society. People stack possessions, knowledge, relationships, degrees, money, jobs, toys, businesses, experiences, etc. They stress, fight, fatigue, compete, become ill, and get anxious and depressed through the process of stacking; yet, few people have found happiness. Society tells us that if our stack is high and mighty, we'll have obtained success. What a deception. What are you stacking; or what do you feel compelled to stack? How were cigarettes supporting that stack?

Allow the stack to fall. This lesson is not encouraging complacency; but instead teaches that real, authentic, and fulfilling work and action can only happen apart from the stress and worry of stacking. When you stack, you're focused on the future and the perceived importance of the stack; and then you have to maintain that heap of nonsense, which requires a lot of anxiety and pressure - by now you know that smoking does not help with that anxiety and pressure. Focus on your experience in the present moment; and if the stack falls, then smile and laugh. Everyone's stack falls, so be healthy and happy when yours does.

*15 minutes of silence and focused breathing. Repeat the mantra: **"I allow the stack to fall."**

(Share this experience using **#30DaysStack**)

<u>Day 21</u>

Exercise:

Think of a major worry that consistently upsets you. On a sheet of paper, write down three worst-case scenarios for that dominating concern. For example, if someone is persistently worried about dying alone, that individual can write as a worst-case scenario, "I will die alone, without anyone at my side, and without family or loved ones to say goodbye." As mentioned, write down three worst-case scenarios for the worry. The worry doesn't have to be as extreme as dying alone; use whichever worry hinders you.

Now, next to each of those three worst-case scenarios write, "I accept this."

Worry is an illness that goes untreated in most people. Think of worry like a cancer of the spirit; but few people know how to treat it effectively. One of the only ways to eradicate worry isn't to fight, ignore, run, or smoke it away; but to face it in the present moment and accept it for the illusion it is. You can never be worried about something happening in the present moment – that's impossible. You can only be worried about the future, which is always illusory.

Writing down your worries and worst-case scenarios, if they ever do come true *(which they rarely do)*, is a great way to draw those thoughts out of your mind and into the present moment, allowing you to face, accept, and observe them without the crutch of cigarettes.

*15 minutes of silence and focused breathing. Repeat the mantra: **"Worries are not real. They are passing thoughts."**

(Share this experience using **#30DaysWorstCase**)

Day 22

Exercise:

Choose a physical symbol that will remind you to observe and be aware in the present moment. Try to choose something from nature, or that is made of natural material.

The object you choose can be anything, but it's best if it's something that you can enjoy looking at and touching. For example, many walkers and hikers will find a unique rock small enough to carry in their hands. A stone, necklace, bracelet, seashell, cedar block, coin…anything will do, as long as you enjoy it and you can dedicate it as a tool for remembrance.

Another cunning trick of cigarettes is to confuse the mind into forgetting you're part of the natural world. Smoking requires you to use hormonal responses, which can be easily manipulated. Thus, when you smoke cigarettes you're taken out of physical reality and put into a false one. It's far better to live aware and awakened in the physical and present moment than experiencing a cigarette.

By having a symbol of remembrance, you can reconnect with the present moment. This symbol isn't meant to be an idol, god, or icon. Don't think too deeply into this. The symbol is simply a tool to help you remember where you are in the *here and now*. As long as you're aware of the present, you'll have no desire to return to the hallucinations manifested by smoking cigarettes.

*15 minutes of silence and focused breathing. Repeat the mantra: **"All is well. Here and now, all is well."**

(Share this experience using **#30DaysSymbol**)

<u>Day 23</u>

Exercise:

Clean something slowly. Take your time; don't rush the cleaning, and be thorough. You can clean your room, car, kitchen, bathroom, bag, desk drawer, shoes…anything. Go slow, and give full attention to what you're doing. Throw away as much stuff as possible.

Most of us hate cleaning and only do it when the mess has become awful; however, cleaning has been known to be a great therapeutic exercise because we attach to our clutter. Regular cleaning is a wonderful practice because we're letting go of disorder in the present moment, in a very practical way.

Similar to a messy kitchen that can look depressing; the mind can experience depression because of thought clutter. Remember that smoking addiction is an illusion, so the person who utilizes cigarettes is filling the mind and body with misconceptions and fantasies that block authentic perception in the present moment. The only way to clear this type of unseemly mental clutter is through observation, understanding, and awareness.

The exercises in this book are purposed to help clear your mind from the mess that a smoking habit leaves behind, so you can perceive clearly. If you haven't experienced it already, waking up to a life without a cigarette dependency is refreshing and exciting.

*15 minutes of silence and focused breathing. Repeat the mantra: **"I am clean. My mind is clear."**

(Share this experience using **#30DaysClean**)

Day 24

Exercise:

On a sheet of paper (one that you can easily save and return to later) make a list of hobbies that you've had in the past but have neglected, and also make a list of hobbies that you would like to start in the future.

From these lists choose one hobby from the past and one new hobby that you'd like to start. Focus only on these two – the old hobby and the new one. Make this a priority.

How often have you said, or have heard other people say, *"I wish I had the time for a hobby."* You do have the time. You just choose to think of time in the way that you've been taught to perceive it. If your life depended on it, you would certainly make the time if needed.

In fact, time is a manmade construct - don't ever forget that. There is only the present moment. Past and future are not here and now. We spend far too much time thinking about time. How many of your recurrent inner thoughts involve questions such as, *"When will that ever happen?" "When will I ever change?" "Why did that have to occur?" "If the past were different, life would be better."*

Smoking occupies the present moment, and that moment could be used to pursue hobbies that magnify your happiness. Think of the time and money saved when you stop smoking - all of those resources can now be put toward growing, rediscovering, and pursuing your hobbies.

*15 minutes of silence and focused breathing. Repeat the mantra: **"The time is now. Happiness is present."**

(Share this experience using **#30DaysHobby**)

<u>Day 25</u>

Exercise:

Hold a smile for 5 minutes. You don't need to do this exercise in front of a mirror, but feel free to do so if you wish. You can even do this exercise during the 15 minutes of silence and focused breathing. While holding your smile, take a moment and feel your face; actually touch the smile and the curvature of your lips and cheekbones.

Have you ever behaved a certain way and then saw your mood change immediately? Physical exercise, such as running and weightlifting, does this for many people. Certain forms of yoga have also been used by people to change their moods. The point is: changing your behavior not only impacts other people, but can also impact your perception of yourself.

You'll notice that while you're smiling during this exercise, you may experience certain emotions. You might feel silly, embarrassed, stupid, funny, weird, or whatever. Continue smiling regardless. Likewise, if you are still thinking about smoking at this point in the program, smile while you're experiencing those thoughts – hold the smile until the thoughts pass; set a reminder alarm if needed. As always, observe your thoughts while you're smiling; observe the thoughts as if they're clouds passing by in a bright blue sky. Smile the adverse thoughts away.

Smiling causes an authentic reaction in our bodies and minds that is essentially good. The present moment enjoys a nice smile. So hold that smile until you no longer can.

*15 minutes of silence and focused breathing. Repeat the mantra: **"Happiness is always now. I am happy."**

(Share this experience using **#30DaysSmile**)

<u>Day 26</u>

Exercise:

Today, look for the color blue in your surrounding environment. If possible, spend the entire day looking for the color blue in the places you go to. Whether you're doing this exercise in a bedroom, office, classroom, outside, or while traveling, look for the color blue in all things that surround you. If you think you'll forget to do this throughout the entire day, spend at least 20 focused minutes practicing this exercise at some point.

Focused attention is something that must be practiced - it doesn't come easy in our rapid-paced society. Instead of encouraging us to focus and observe, the modern world encourages us to rush and get things done.

Searching for a color or shape helps to slow down our accelerated and cyclical thought patterns, and reminds us that there's more to the world than the chaotic thoughts we collectively and daily experience. By searching for the color blue, your mind can escape the fictitious grip of anxiety, lust, desire, depression, worry, fear, or any other potent emotion. When you were smoking, were you aware of the stunning colors around you? Most likely not.

Smoking functions to distract your conscience from present reality. Look for the color blue today, and wake up to life in the present moment.

*15 minutes of silence and focused breathing. Repeat the mantra: **"I am focused, here and now."**

(Share this experience using **#30DaysBlue**)

Day 27

Exercise:

Go for a mindfulness walk for at least 10 minutes. Focus on each step. Feel the steps: the feel of your feet hitting the ground, your heel rolling forward, your toes, the bend of your knees, your hips working to balance your posture, the swinging of your arms, etc. Don't rush; go slow. Focus on your breathing as well. Get in tune with your body. Pay attention to your physical senses throughout the walk. Focus – don't listen to music or be distracted.

Human beings have always used walking as a naturally restorative exercise. There is something about walking, and focusing on the walk, that calms the mind and soul. The longer one walks, the more relaxed one feels.

Any moment is a good time to walk and experience your inner and outer environment. During long walks, thoughts will emerge that will allow you to consciously observe them. Let the thoughts pass; you may even have emotions that emerge, observe those and let them pass as well. Focusing on your steps will help you clear the mind of clutter. Walking in the early morning and at dusk is especially beneficial.

A 20-minute walk brings more comfort, stillness, peace, focus, and awareness than thousands of hours of smoking cigarettes. Walk every day, as much as you can.

*15 minutes of silence and focused breathing. Repeat the mantra: **"I am relaxed. I am at peace."**

(Share this experience using **#30DaysWalk**)

<u>Day 28</u>

Exercise:

With eyes closed, feel your heartbeat for two to three minutes. Don't count the beats; instead, get in tune with its rhythm. Also, don't try to change its rhythm. Continue to breathe normally. You can feel your heart's beat by placing two fingers on the side of your neck just under your jawbone (carotid pulse), placing a hand on your chest (bronchial pulse), or placing two fingers on the inside of your wrist (radial pulse). Use whichever method gives you the best feeling of your heart's beat. Let your thoughts go, and focus entirely on the rhythm of your heart beating.

We can live our entire lives completely unaware that there is an engineering marvel in our chest. Think about it. Your heart started beating when you were in the womb, it has been beating ever since, and it will continue to beat until you leave this blue planet. It is an amazing pump that does not stop until it's our time to experience death. The heart slows down to rest, but it never takes a break. Experience your magnificent heart, and get in tune with its rhythm.

Similar to listening to your breathing, feeling your heart's rhythm during meditation can help you gain present moment awareness. Be aware of your heart, know its rhythm, treat it well, be thankful for its endurance and strength, and let it beat. If you're ever stressed, don't consider smoking; instead, remember your breath and heartbeat. Why continue smoking a toxin that damages your amazing heart? Let your heart beat healthily.

*15 minutes of silence and focused breathing. Repeat the mantra: ***"My heart is strong and gives me life."***

(Share this experience using **#30DaysHeart**)

<u>Day 29</u>

Exercise:

Make yourself laugh for 5 minutes. Don't stop laughing. You might feel strange, weird, embarrassed, or stupid…it doesn't matter, just laugh. Try to laugh alone and without the aid of a comedy or joke. If you don't know how to start, just start making the noises that typically accompany your laughter.

What feelings did you experience during this exercise? Many people report feeling embarrassed or goofy, which is great; however, most people also report a feeling of relief and buoyancy when they've completed this exercise.

Similar to holding a smile, laughing for 5 minutes is a fantastic way to come into present awareness. If you think about it, humor is necessary for life. How sad is the person who is unable to laugh at the experiences of life? After all, life is funny, even the dreadful and lousy experiences.

Laughter is a way to relax, open up, become carefree, and allow yourself to be at peace with all of your perceived faults, adverse habits, and struggles. When you laugh, even to the point of tears, you strip all the old beliefs of self at that moment and simply enjoy being free from smoking.

Many people attempt to stop using cigarettes by following a "serious" approach to quitting. It's much more beneficial to be balanced by understanding the seriousness of cigarettes' deadly effects on the body, mind, and soul, yet also amusing yourself with the absurdity of the attachment.

*15 minutes of silence and focused breathing. Repeat the mantra: **"Life is wonderful, funny, and real."**

(Share this experience using **#30DaysLaugh**)

Day 30

Exercise:

Take a piece of paper (one that you can keep) and write down all that you are grateful for – these things don't have to be in any particular order of importance.

Next to each thing you list, write "Thank you."

The person who isn't thankful for all that life gives is typically quite miserable, and false self-beliefs thrive on that negativity. The truly grateful person can let go of anything at anytime. A thankful person is always a happy person, so practice gratitude daily. Let your healthy self be...thankful.

Have you ever heard anyone say, *"I am so grateful for cigarettes and all that they have done for me"*? Nobody is thankful for cigarettes' effect on their lives; which is a clear sign that smoking isn't only a danger but also an unwanted societal custom. However, a few people have learned to be thankful for the lessons learned through their negatives experiences with smoking a deadly toxin. Be thankful that you're aware, and be thankful for every moment experienced on this beautiful blue planet.

Not only is it poisonous, but an attachment to smoking cigarettes discourages a grateful mind and soul. With only one life to live in the present moment, it's important to always emphasize a grateful and healthy heart. Spend time with people who are grateful, and do things that nourish a thankful heart in the present moment. Be thankful.

*15 minutes of silence and focused breathing. Repeat the mantra: **"I am grateful. I am thankful. I am healthy."**

(Share this experience using **#30DaysThanks**)

Conclusion

The exercises and lessons in this program taught and encouraged observation, awareness of your present moment experience, change of perception, and awakening to true happiness, which can only be found here and now. You were shown that negative thoughts and feelings about cigarettes are solely within you and illusory; which means that you are capable of letting those thoughts and feelings pass and dropping an attachment to cigarettes in the present moment.

As mentioned at the beginning, there were no goals or measures of success for this program. If you were hoping to find a magical way to stop smoking, then you may be spending too much time struggling and thinking about cigarettes. This was not meant to be a struggle or fight, but a release. You don't need to gain freedom from old beliefs about smoking; you already have it. You were never dependent on cigarettes...you only believed you were.

Life is not meant to be spent fighting an adverse attachment to cigarettes, or any type of unhealthy dependency. Wake up to the present moment and enjoy your present experience. If you've made it through the program, you are certainly more awakened then when you started; however, don't give up mindfully practicing observation of thoughts and feelings, stillness, silence, deep and focused breathing, allowing everything to pass, laughing, smiling, and being grateful.

Live wonderfully awakened, healthy, and aware...without cigarettes influencing your true being. Smoking, or any toxic habit that impacts your physical and mental state, cannot match the power and essence of your awakened self.

www.ingramcontent.com/pod-product-compliance
Lightning Source LLC
Chambersburg PA
CBHW021407160726
47994CB00007B/3109